The Ultimate

Learn Everything You Need .... and
Improve Your Meals with Easy and Tasty Recipes

Tim Singhapat

Table of contents

STEAMED COCONUT CAKES

Ingredients:

- ¼ cup all-purpose flour
- ½ cup coconut milk
- ½ cup grated sweet coconut
- ½ cup rice flour
- 4 tablespoons finely granulated sugar
- 5 eggs
- Pinch of salt

Directions:

1. In a big mixing container, beat the eggs and the sugar together until thick and pale in color.

2. Put in the rice flours and salt.

3. Beating continuously, slowly pour in the coconut milk. Beat the batter for 3 more minutes.

4. Bring some water to boil in a steamer big enough to hold 10 small ramekins. When the water starts to boil, put the ramekins in the steamer to heat for a couple of minutes.

5. Split the shredded coconut uniformly between all of the ramekins and use a spoon to compact it on the bottom of the cups.

6. Pour the batter uniformly between the cups. Steam for about ten minutes.

7. Take away the cakes from the cups the moment they are sufficiently cool to handle.

8. Serve warm or at room temperature.

Yield: 10 cakes

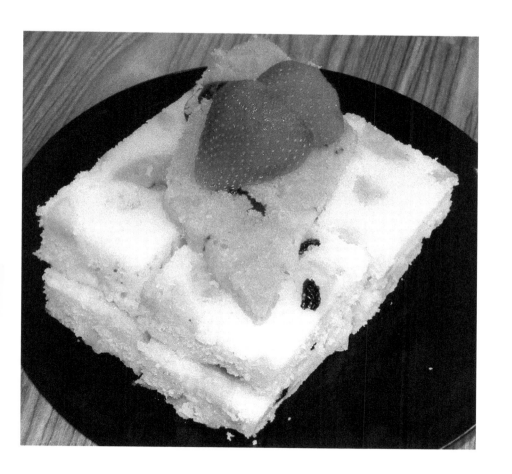

STICKY RICE WITH COCONUT CREAM SAUCE

Ingredients:

- 1 cup coconut cream

- 1 teaspoon salt

- 3 cups cooked Sweet Sticky Rice

- 4 ripe mangoes, thinly cut (or other tropical fruits)

- 4 tablespoons sugar

Directions:

1. For the sauce, put the coconut cream, sugar, and salt in a small deep cooking pan. Stir to blend and bring to its boiling point on moderate to high heat. Decrease the heat and simmer for five minutes.

2. To serve, position mango slices on each plate. Put a mound of rice next to the fruit. Top the rice with some of the sauce.

Yield: Servings 6

SWEET STICKY RICE

Ingredients:

- ½ cup granulated sugar

- ½ teaspoon salt

- 1 cups canned coconut milk

- 1½ cups white glutinous rice

Directions:

1. Put the rice in a container and put in enough water to completely cover the rice. Soak for minimum 4 hours or overnight. Drain.

2. Coat a steamer basket with wet cheesecloth. Spread the rice uniformly over the cheesecloth. Put the container over quickly boiling water. Cover and steam until soft, approximately twenty-five minutes; set aside.

3. In a moderate-sized-sized deep cooking pan, mix the coconut milk, sugar, and salt and heat on moderate to high. Stir until the sugar is thoroughly blended. Pour over the rice, stir until blended, and allow to rest for half an hour

4. To serve, place in small bowls or on plates. Decorate using mangoes, papayas, or other tropical fruit.

Yield: Servings 6

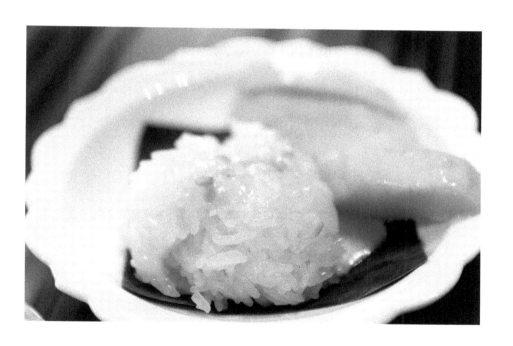

TARO BALLS POACHED IN COCONUT MILK

Ingredients:

- 1 cup brown sugar

- 1 cup cooked taro, mashed

- 1 cup corn flour

- 2 cups glutinous rice flour

- 4 cups coconut milk

- Fresh tropical fruit (not necessary)

- teaspoon salt

Directions:

1. In a big mixing container, mix the rice and the flours.

2. Put in the mashed taro and knead to make a tender dough.

3. Roll into little bite-sized balls and save for later.

4. In a moderate-sized to big deep cooking pan, heat the coconut milk using low heat.

5. Put in the brown sugar and the salt, stirring until blended.

6. Bring the mixture to a low boil and put in the taro balls.

7. Poach the balls for five to ten minutes or until done to your preference.

8. Serve hot in small glass bowls, decorated with tropical fruit.

Yield: Servings 6–12

TOFU WITH SWEET GINGER

Ingredients:

- 1 (2- to 3-inch) piece of ginger, peeled and smashed using the back of a knife

- 1 12-ounce package tender tofu

- 3 cups water

- 1 cup brown sugar

Directions:

1. Put the water, ginger, and brown sugar in a small deep cooking pan. Bring to its boiling point using high heat. Lower the heat to a simmer and allow the sauce to cook for minimum ten minutes. (The longer you allow the mixture to cook, the spicier it will get.)

2. To serve, spoon some of the tofu into dessert bowls and pour some sauce over the top. (This sauce is equally good over plain yogurt.)

Yield: 3 cups of sauce

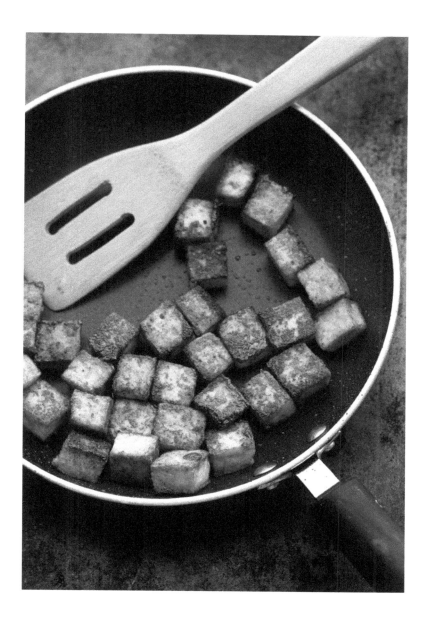

TROPICAL COCONUT RICE

Ingredients:

- ¼ cup toasted coconut

- 1 cup coconut cream

- 2 cups short-grained rice

- 2 cups water

Directions:

1. Place the rice, water, and coconut cream in a moderate-sized deep cooking pan and mix thoroughly. Bring to its boiling point on moderate to high heat. Decrease the heat and cover with a tight-fitting lid. Cook for fifteen to twenty minutes or until all of the liquid has been absorbed.

2. Allow the rice rest off the heat for five minutes.

3. Fluff the rice and mix in the toasted coconut and fruit.

Yield: Servings 6–8

TROPICAL FRUIT WITH GINGER CREÈME ANGLAISE

Ingredients:

- (1-inch) pieces peeled gingerroot, slightly mashed 1
- cup half-and-half

- 2 tablespoons sugar A variety of tropical fruits, cut

- 3 egg yolks

Directions:

1. In a small heavy deep cooking pan on moderate to low heat, bring the ginger and the half-and-half to a slight simmer. Do not boil.

2. Meanwhile, whisk together the eggs yolks and the sugar.

3. Slowly pour the hot half-and-half into the egg mixture, stirring continuously so that the eggs do not cook.

4. Pour the custard back into the deep cooking pan and cook on moderate to low heat, stirring continuously using a wooden spoon for five minutes or until slightly thickened.

5. Pour the crèmes anglaise through a mesh strainer into a clean container and let cool completely.

6. Pour over slices of your favorite tropical fruits.

Yield: 1½ cups

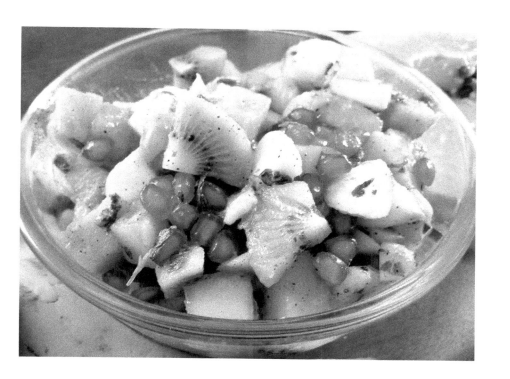

WATERMELON ICE

Ingredients:

- ½ cup sugar

- 1 (3-pound) piece of watermelon, rind cut away, seeded, and cut into little chunks (reserve a small amount for decoration if you wish)

- 1 cup water

- 1 tablespoon lime juice

- Mint sprigs (not necessary)

Directions:

1. Put the water and sugar in a small deep cooking pan and bring to its boiling point. Turn off the heat and let cool to room temperature, stirring regularly. Set the pan in a container of ice and continue to stir the syrup until cold.

2. Put the watermelon, syrup, and lime juice in a blender and puréee until the desired smoothness is achieved.

3. Pour the puréee through a sieve into a 9-inch baking pan. Cover the pan using foil.

4. Put into your freezer the purée for eight hours or until frozen.

5. To serve, scrape the frozen purée with the tines of a fork. Ladle the scrapings into pretty glass goblets and decorate with a small piece of watermelon or mint sprigs.

Yield: Servings 6–8

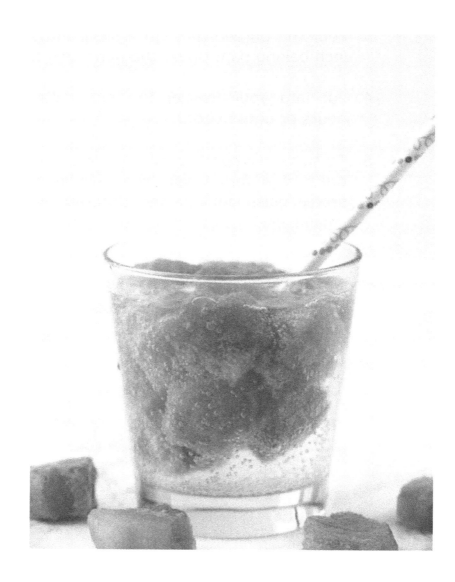

FRESH COCONUT JUICE

Ingredients:

- 1 young coconut

- Ice

- Sprig of mint for decoration

Directions:

1. Using a meat cleaver, make a V-shaped slice on the top of the coconut.

2. Pour the juice over a glass of ice.

3. Decorate using a mint sprig.

Yield: Servings 1–2 depending on the size of the coconut.

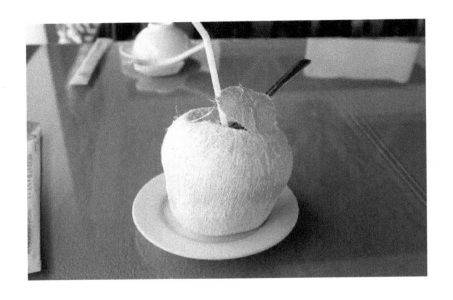

GINGER TEA

Ingredients:

- ½-¾ cup sugar

- 1 big branch (roughly

- 8 cups water

- pound) of ginger, cut into long pieces

Directions:

1. Bring the water to its boiling point in a big pan. Put in the ginger, reduce heat, and simmer for ten to twenty minutes, depending on how strong you prefer your tea.

2. Take away the ginger and put in the sugar to taste, stirring until it is thoroughly blended.

3. Serve hot or over ice.

Yield: 8 cups

ICED SWEET TEA

Ingredients:

- 1 cup hot water

- 1 tablespoon sugar

- 1 tablespoon sweetened condensed milk

- 1 teaspoon milk

- 1–2 tablespoons Thai tea leaves

- Ice

Directions:

1. Place the sugar and sweetened condensed milk into a big glass.

2. Put the tea leaves into a tea ball and place it in the glass.

3. Put in the hot water. Allow to steep until done to your preferred strength.

4. Stir to dissolve the sugar and sweetened condensed milk.

5. Put in ice and top with milk.

Yield: slightly more than 1 cup.

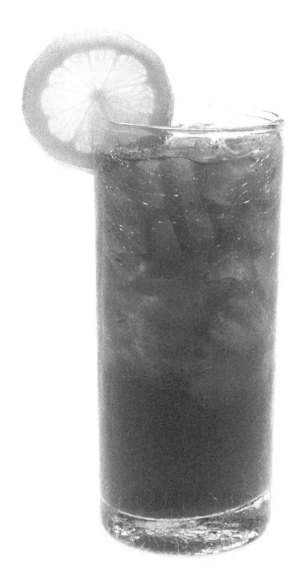

LEMONGRASS TEA

Ingredients:

- ¼– cup sugar

- 1 cup lemongrass stalks, chopped

- 8 cups water

Directions:

1. Bring the water to its boiling point in a big pan. Put in the lemongrass, turn off the heat, and allow to steep for ten to twenty minutes, depending on how strong you prefer your tea.

2. Take away the lemongrass and put in the sugar to taste, stirring until it is thoroughly blended.

3. Serve hot or over ice.

Yield: 8 cups

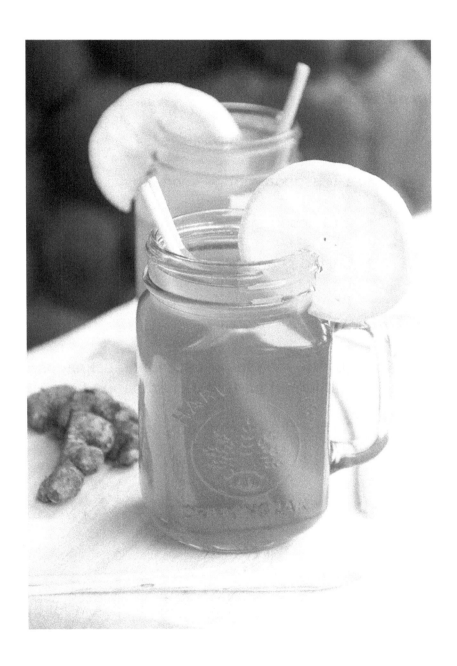

MANGO BELLINI

Ingredients:

- ½ teaspoon lemon juice

- 1 teaspoon mango schnapps

- 2 tablespoons puréed mango

- Chilled champagne

Directions:

1. Put the mango purée, mango schnapps, and lemon juice in a champagne flute.

2. Fill the flute with champagne and stir.

Yield: 1 glass

ROYAL THAI KIR

Ingredients:

- 1–2 teaspoons creème de mango or mango schnapps Chilled dry
- champagne

Directions:

1. Pour the creème into a champagne flute and fill with champagne.

Yield: 1 glass

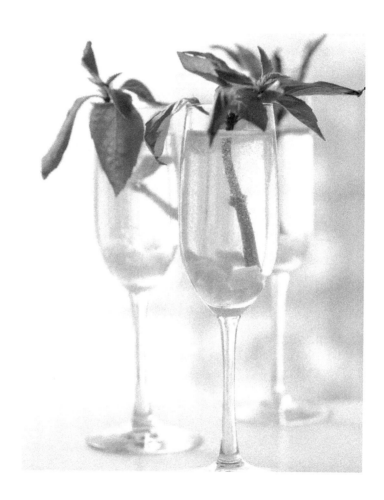

SUPER-SIMPLE THAI ICED TEA

Ingredients:

- 2 tablespoons sugar

- 1 cup hot water

- Ice

- 1–2 tablespoons Thai tea leaves

Directions:

1. Place the sugar into a big glass.

2. Put the tea leaves in a tea ball and place it in the glass.

3. Put in the hot water. Allow to steep until done to your preferred strength.

4. Stir to dissolve the sugar and put in ice.

Yield: Approximately 1 cup

THAI "MARTINIS"

Ingredients:

- 1 bottle coconut rum

- 1 bottle dark rum

- 1 bottle light rum

- 1 whole ripe pineapple

- 3 stalks lemongrass, trimmed, cut into 3-inch lengths and tied in a bundle

Directions:

1. Take away the pineapple greens and then quarter the rest of the fruit. Put the pineapple quarters and the lemongrass bundle in a container big enough to hold all of the liquor.

2. Pour the rums over the fruit and stir until blended. Cover the container and let

infuse for minimum one week at room temperature.

3. Take away the lemongrass bundle and discard.

4. Take away the pineapple quarters and slice into slices for decoration.

5. To serve, pour some of the rum into a martini shaker filled with ice; shake thoroughly. Pour into martini glasses and decorate with a pineapple slice.

Yield: 3 quarts

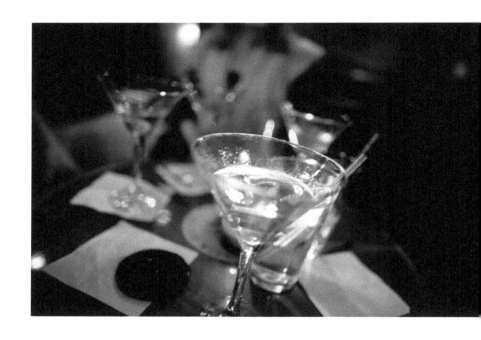

THAI ICED TEA

Ingredients:

- 1 cup sugar

- 1 cup Thai tea leaves

- 1–1½ cups half-and-half

- 6 cups water

- Ice

Directions:

1. Bring the water to boil in a moderate-sized pot. Turn off the heat and put in the tea leaves, pushing them into the water until they are completely submerged. Steep roughly five minutes or until the liquid is a bright orange.

2. Strain through a fine-mesh sieve or coffee strainer.

3. Mix in the sugar until thoroughly blended.

4. Allow the tea to reach room temperature and then place in your fridge

5. To serve, pour the tea over ice cubes, leaving room at the top of the glass to pour in three to 4 tablespoons of half-and-half; stir for a short period of time to blend.

Yield: Approximately 8 cups

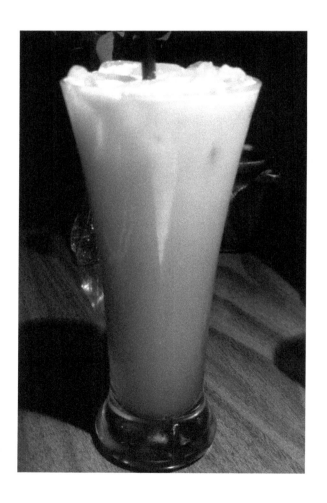

THAI LIMEADE

Ingredients:

- 1–½ cup sugar

- 1 cup lime juice, lime rinds reserved

- 8 cups water

- Salt to taste (not necessary)

Directions:

1. Mix the lime juice and the sugar; set aside.

2. Bring the water to boil in a big pot. Put in the lime rinds and turn off the heat. Allow to steep for ten to fifteen minutes. Take away the lime rinds.

3. Put in the lime juice mixture to the hot water, stirring to completely dissolve the sugar. Put in salt if you wish.

4. Serve over ice.

Yield: 9 cups

THAI-INSPIRED SINGAPORE SLING

Ingredients:

- ¼– cup pineapple juice Mint sprig (not necessary)

- 1 tablespoon cherry brandy

- 1 tablespoon lime juice

- 1 tablespoon orange liqueur

- 1 teaspoon brown sugar

- 2 tablespoons whiskey

- Dash of bitters

Directions:

1. Put all of the ingredients into a cocktail shaker and shake thoroughly to blend.

2. Serve over crushed ice and decorate with a sprig of mint if you wish.

Yield: 1 cocktail

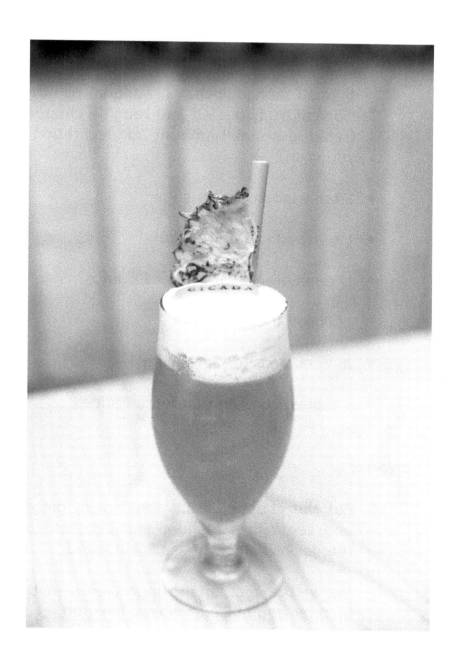

TROPICAL FRUIT COCKTAIL

Ingredients:

- 1 small mango, papaya, banana, or other tropical fruit, peeled and roughly chopped (reserve a small amount for decoration if you wish)

- 1 tablespoon brown sugar

- 1 teaspoon grated ginger

- 1/ cups orange or grapefruit juice

- 1/ cups pineapple juice

- 1–½ cup (or to taste) rum

- 4 tablespoons lime or lemon juice

Directions:

1. Put the chopped fruit, lime juice, ginger, and sugar in a blender and process until the desired smoothness is achieved.

2. Put in the rest of the ingredients to the blender and pulse until well blended.

3. To serve, pour over crushed ice and garnish with fruit slices of your choice.

Yield: 3–4 cups

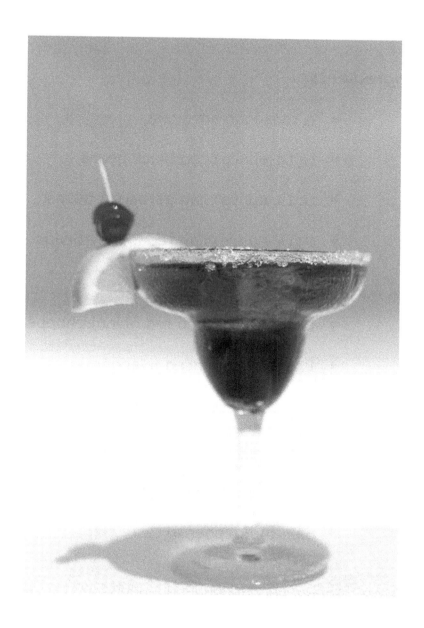

ASIAN 3-BEAN SALAD

Ingredients:

- ½ teaspoon lime zest

- 1 (14-ounce) can black beans

- 1 (14-ounce) can garbanzo beans

- 1 (14-ounce) can red kidney beans

- 1 cup chopped cilantro

- 1 moderate-sized red onion, chopped

- 1 teaspoon minced jalapeño

- 3 cloves garlic, minced

- 3 tablespoons rice vinegar

- 4 tablespoons olive oil

- Salt and pepper to taste

Directions:

1. Put all the beans in a colander. Thoroughly wash under cool running water. Drain and save for later.

2. Mix together all the rest of the ingredients and pour over beans; stir until blended.

3. Place in your fridge overnight, stirring once in a while. Sprinkle with salt and pepper.

Yield: Servings 4–6

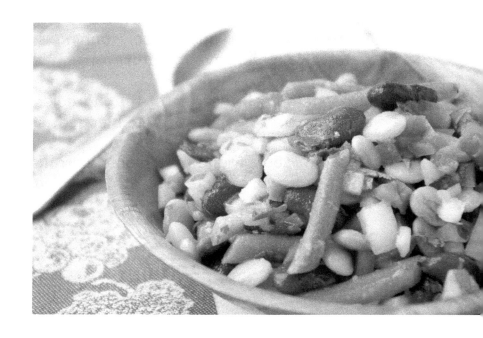

ASIAN CARROT STICKS

Ingredients:

- −¼ teaspoon cayenne pepper

- ½–½ teaspoons paprika

- ½–1 teaspoon Chinese 5-spice powder

- 1 pound thin carrots, peeled and slice into quarters along the length

- 2 cloves garlic, minced

- 2 tablespoons rice vinegar

- 3 tablespoons chopped cilantro

- 4 tablespoons olive oil

- 4 tablespoons water

- Salt and pepper to taste

Directions:

1. Put the carrots in a pan big enough to hold them easily.

2. Cover the carrots with water and bring to its boiling point using high heat. Drain the carrots and return them to the pan.

3. Put in the 4 tablespoons of water, the olive oil, and the garlic; bring to its boiling point, reduce to a simmer, and cook until just soft. Drain.

4. In a small container, mix together rest of the ingredients; pour over the carrots, tossing to coat.

5. Sprinkle salt and pepper to taste.

6. The carrots may be eaten instantly, but develop a richer flavor if allowed to marinate for a few hours.

Yield: Servings 4–6

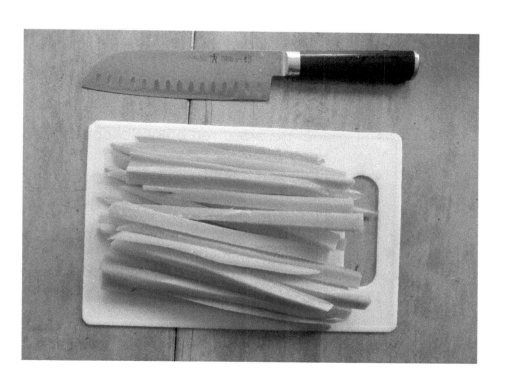

ASIAN COUSCOUS SALAD

Ingredients:

- ½ cup vegetable oil

- 1 clove garlic, minced

- 1 moderate-sized red onion, chopped

- 1 packed cup basil

- 1 packed cup cilantro

- 1 packed cup mint

- 1 pound snow peas, trimmed

- 1 red bell pepper, cored, seeded, and chopped

- 1 yellow bell pepper, cored, seeded, and chopped 1–2 jalapeño chilies, seeded and
- finely chopped 2 tablespoons
- lemon juice 2¾ cups
- couscous

- 3 tablespoons lime juice

- 3½ cups boiling water, divided

5–7 green onions, trimmed and thinly cut
- Salt and freshly ground
- black pepper to taste

Directions:

1. Put the snow peas, peppers, onions, chilies, garlic, and couscous in a big container; toss to blend.

2. Pour 3 cups of the boiling water over the couscous mixture, cover firmly, and allow it to stand at room temperature for an hour.

3. Put in the remaining fi cup boiling water and all the rest of the ingredients to the couscous; toss together, cover, and allow it to stand for minimum 30 more minutes.

4. Sprinkle with salt and freshly ground black pepper.

Yield: Servings 8–10

ASIAN MARINARA SAUCE

Ingredients:

- 1 (1-inch) piece of ginger, peeled and minced

- 1 cup water

- 1 medium onion, chopped

- 1 pound chopped canned tomatoes with the juice

- 1 teaspoon salt

- 1 teaspoon sugar

- 1—3 serrano chilies, seeded and minced 2 tablespoons
- vegetable oil

Directions:

1. In a big deep cooking pan, heat the oil or moderate heat.

2. Put in the onion and ginger and sauté for a couple of minutes.

3. Put in the chilies and carry on cooking one minute more.

4. Mix in the water, tomatoes, salt, and sugar. Decrease the heat to low and simmer for minimum 30 minutes.

Yield: Approximately 2 cups

ASIAN RATATOUILLE

Ingredients:

- ½ teaspoon salt

- ½-inch cubes

- ¾ cup vegetable stock

- 1 cup cut mushrooms

- 1 onion, slivered

- 1 red bell pepper, cored, seeded, and julienned

- 1 tablespoon chopped cilantro

- 1 tablespoon cornstarch

- 1 tablespoon dry sherry

- 1 teaspoon minced garlic

- 1 teaspoon minced ginger

- 2 Japanese eggplants (approximately 1 pound), cut into

- 2 ribs of celery, cut

- 2 small zucchini, halved along the length and cut

- 2 tablespoons soy sauce

- 2 teaspoons <u>Plum Dipping Sauce (Page 34)</u>

- 3 tablespoons sesame oil

- 3 tablespoons vegetable oil

Directions:

1. Put the eggplant in a colander and drizzle with the salt. Allow to rest for half an hour

2. In a big ovenproof pot, heat the sesame oil on medium. Put in the celery, onion, and red bell pepper; sautée for five minutes. Take the vegetables out of the pan and save for later.

3. Put in the vegetable oil to the pot. Sauté the zucchini, mushrooms, and eggplant for five minutes. Mix in the celery, onion, and bell pepper and save for later.

4. In a small mixing container, whisk together the stock, soy sauce, sherry, and cornstarch. Pour over the vegetables and stir until blended.

5. Bake, covered, in a 350-degree oven for forty minutes.

6. Mix in the garlic, ginger, and plum sauce. Cover and carry on baking for another ten minutes.

Yield: Servings 6–8

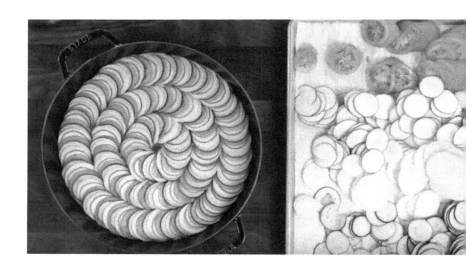

ASIAN-INSPIRED CHICKEN AND WILD RICE SOUP

Ingredients:

- 1 tablespoon vegetable oil

- 1–2 garlic cloves, minced

- 2 tablespoons fish sauce

- 2 whole boneless, skinless chicken breasts, trimmed and slice into fine strips

- 2–3 teaspoons minced ginger

- 6 cups low-fat, low-salt chicken broth

Directions:

1. In a big soup pot, heat the oil on moderate to high. Put in the chicken strips and sauté for two to three minutes.

2. Put in the garlic and gingerroot and sauté for one more minute.
3. Mix in the fish sauce, broth, and rice. Bring to its boiling point; reduce heat, cover, and simmer for about ten minutes.

4. Put in the green onions and snow peas; simmer to heat through.

5. Adjust seasoning with salt and freshly ground white pepper to taste.

Yield: Servings 6–8

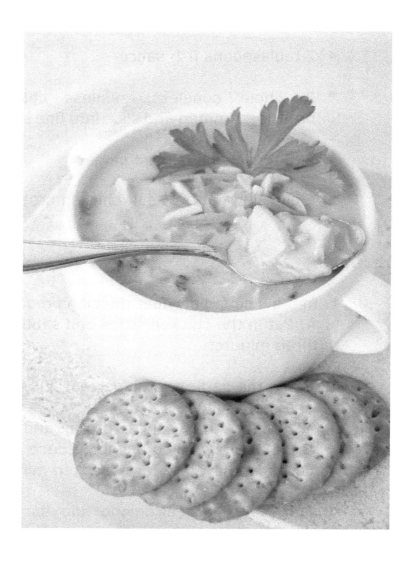

CHICKEN SALAD 1

Ingredients:

For the dressing:

- ¼ cup vegetable oil
- ½; teaspoon (or to taste) salt
- 1 tablespoon soy sauce
- 2 tablespoons rice wine vinegar
- 2 teaspoons grated gingerroot
- Pinch of sugar

For the salad:

- 1 cup bean sprouts
- 1 medium head of Chinese cabbage, shredded
- 1 tablespoon toasted sesame seeds
- 2 cups chopped cooked chicken
- 3 green onions, trimmed and cut

- 4 ounces snow peas, trimmed

Directions:

1. Put the salad dressing ingredients in a small container and whisk vigorously to blend.

2. In a moderate-sized-sized container, mix the chicken, snow peas, green onions, and bean sprouts. Put in the dressing and toss to coat.

3. To serve, position the cabbage on a serving platter. Mound the chicken salad over the cabbage. Decorate using the sesame seeds.

Yield: Servings 4

CHICKEN SALAD 2

Ingredients:

- ¼ cup chopped cilantro, plus extra for decoration

- ¼ pound rice sticks

- 1 cup cut scallions

- 1 tablespoon dry sherry

- 1 tablespoon soy sauce

- 1 tablespoon vegetable oil

- 1 teaspoon sesame oil

- 2 whole boneless, skinless chicken breasts

- 3 tablespoons hoisin sauce, divided

- 3 tablespoons peanuts, chopped

- 3 tablespoons sesame seeds, toasted

- 4 tablespoons lime juice

- Bibb or romaine lettuce leaves

- Peanut oil for frying

Directions:

1. Mix 1 tablespoon of the hoisin sauce, the soy sauce, and the sherry in a moderate-sized container. Put in the chicken breasts and marinate for twenty minutes to half an hour.

2. Heat the vegetable oil in a big frying pan on moderate to high heat. Put in the chicken breasts, saving for later the marinade. Brown the breasts on both sides. Put in the reserved marinade to the frying pan, cover, and cook on moderate to low heat until soft, approximately twenty minutes.

3. Allow the chicken to cool completely, then shred it into bite-sized pieces; set aside.

4. In a moderate-sized-sized container, mix the shredded chicken with the rest of the hoisin sauce, the lime juice, sesame oil, sesame seeds, peanuts, scallions, and cilantro. Put in the shredded chicken and stir to coat.

5. Put in roughly an inch of peanut oil to a big frying pan and heat on high until the oil is super hot, but not smoking.

6. Put in the rice sticks cautiously and fry for roughly 6 to 8 seconds or until puffed and golden; turn the rice sticks using tongs and fry for another 6 to 8 seconds. Take away the rice sticks to a stack of paper towels to drain.

7. Toss about of the rice sticks with the chicken mixture.

8. To serve, place a mound of salad on a lettuce leaf on the center of each plate. Top with the rest of the rice sticks and decorate with additional cilantro.

Yield: Servings 4–6

CHICKEN SALAD 3

Ingredients:

- ½ cup soy sauce

- ½ cup super slimly cut celery

- ½ teaspoon sesame oil (not necessary)

- 1 (¼-inch) piece ginger, peeled and minced

- 1 clove garlic, minced

- 1 cup cooked chicken meat

- 1 scallion, thinly cut

- 1 tablespoon sugar

- 1 teaspoon vegetable oil

- 2 tablespoons rice vinegar

- cups shredded bok choy

Directions:

1. In a moderate-sized-sized container, toss together the chicken, bok choy, celery, and scallion.

2. In a small container, meticulously whisk together the rest of the ingredients. Pour over the salad and toss thoroughly to blend.

Yield: 3–4 cups

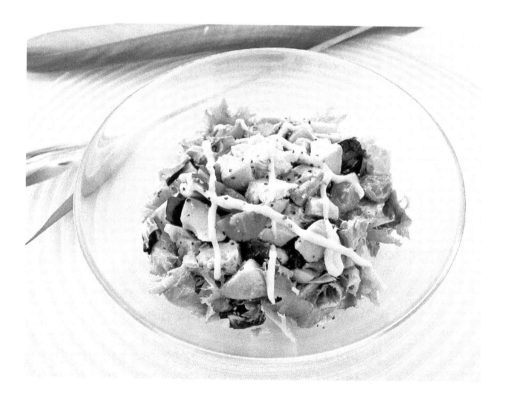

CRAZY COCONUT PIE

Ingredients:

- ½ cup flour

- ¾ cup sugar

- ¾ stick of butter, melted

- 1 cup sweetened shredded coconut

- 1½ teaspoons vanilla

- 2 cups milk

- 4 eggs

Directions:

1. Preheat your oven to 350 degrees. Grease and flour a 10-inch pie plate.

2. Put all of the ingredients in a blender and blend for a minute. Pour the batter into the readied pan.

3. Bake for about forty-five minutes or until golden on top.

Yield: 1 (10-inch) pie

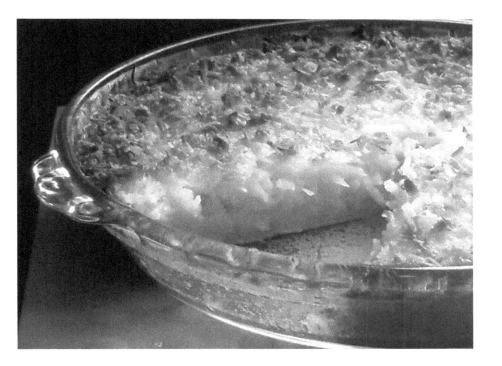

CREAM OF COCONUT CRABMEAT DIP

Ingredients:

- ¼ teaspoon salt 2 green onions, trimmed and thinly cut ¾ cup cream of coconut

- 1 jalapeño, seeded and minced

- 1 tablespoon lemon or lime juice

- 1¼ pounds (10 ounces) crabmeat, picked over to remove shell pieces

- 2 tablespoons chopped cilantro

- Ground white pepper to taste

Directions:

1. In a small deep cooking pan, mix the cream of coconut, crabmeat, and salt; bring to a simmer on moderate to low heat. Simmer for five minutes.

2. Mix in the green onions, cilantro, lemon juice, jalapeño, and pepper. Pour into a serving dish and allow it to stand at room temperature until cool.

3. Serve with fresh vegetables and crackers.

Yield: Approximately 2 cups

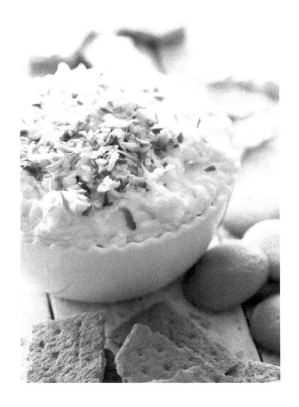

CRUNCHY SPROUT SALAD

Ingredients:

- ¼ cup rice vinegar

- 1 tablespoon sugar

- 2 cups sprouts of your choice

- 2 tablespoons fish or soy sauce

- 2 tablespoons vegetable oil

- 2 teaspoons grated gingerroot

- 6 cups baby greens (if possible an Asian mix

Directions:

1. In a big container whisk together the vinegar fish sauce, vegetable oil, sugar, and gingerroot.

2. Put in the sprouts, toss to coat, and le marinate for half an hour
3. Put in the greens and toss until well blended

Yield: Servings 4

GRILLED LOBSTER TAILS WITH A LEMONGRASS SMOKE

Ingredients:

- 3–4 whole lemongrass stalks, bruised

- 6 (4–6 ounce) lobster tails

- Cracked black pepper

- Olive oil

- Salt to taste

Directions:

1. To prepare the lobster tails, lay each tail flat-side down (shell up). Using a sharp knife, cut through the shell and midway through the meat along the length. Use your fingers to pull the meat away from the membranes and the inner shell, then invert the meat until it sits on top of the shell instead of being surrounded by it.

2. Brush the lobster liberally with olive oil and drizzle with black pepper. Put the lemongrass stalks in a Tuscan herb grill.
3. Heat grill to moderate-high heat. Put the herb grill on the main grill grate and put the lobster tails on top, meat side up. Close the lid of the grill and cook for seven to eight minutes. (The shells must be bright red and the meat fairly firm.)

4. Flip the lobster tails over and carry on cooking for two to three minutes.

5. Drizzle with salt before you serve.

Yield: Servings 6

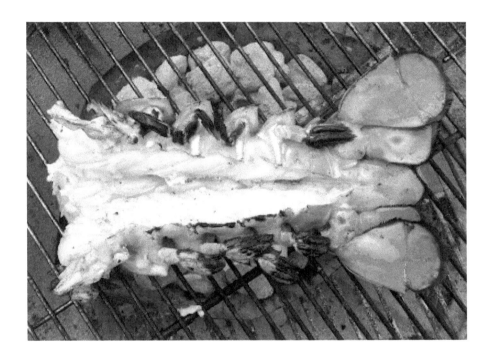

GRILLED STEAK WITH PEANUT SAUCE

Ingredients:

- 1 (2-pound) flank steak, trimmed

- 1 recipe of Peanut Dipping Sauce

- 1 recipe of Thai Marinade

Directions:

1. Swiftly wash the steak under cold water and pat dry. Put the steak in a big Ziplock bag together with the marinade. Flip the meat until it is thoroughly coated with the marinade on all sides. Place in your fridge overnight.(Allow the steak return to room temperature before cooking.)

2. Preheat a broiler or grill. Cook the steak, flipping over once and coating with the rest of the marinade, until done to your preference

3. Take away the meat from the grill, cover it using foil, and allow it to rest for five minutes to let some of the juices reabsorb. To serve, finely slice the steak across the grain. Pass the peanut sauce separately.

Yield: Servings 6

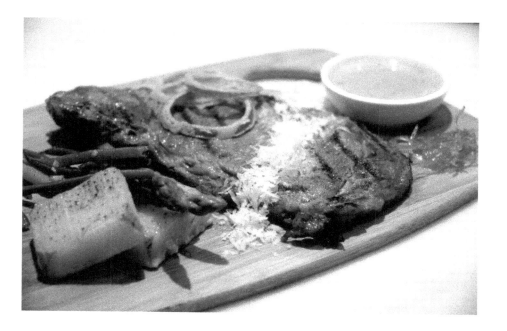

JICAMA, CARROT, AND CHINESE CABBAGE SALAD

Ingredients:

- ½ cup chopped cilantro

- ½ teaspoon prepared chili-garlic sauce

- 1 cup vegetable oil

- 1 teaspoon ground anise

- 2 big carrots, peeled and finely julienned

- 2 pounds jicama, peeled and finely julienned

- 2 tablespoons lime juice

- 3/4 pound Chinese cabbage, thinly shredded Salt and black
- pepper to taste

Directions:

1. Thoroughly mix the ground anise, cilantro, vegetable oil, lime juice, and chili-garlic sauce in a big mixing container.

2. Put in the vegetables and toss to coat.

3. Sprinkle with salt and pepper.

Yield: Servings 6–8

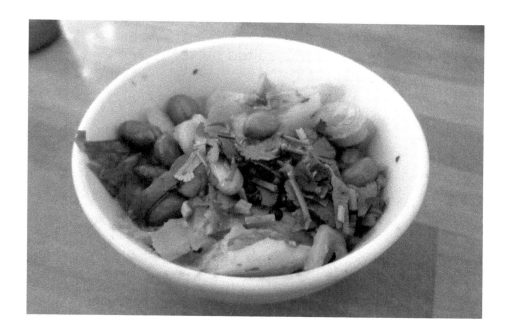

LIME BUTTER CAKE

Ingredients:

- ¼ teaspoon salt

- 1 cup milk

- 1½ cups sugar

- 2 sticks unsalted butter

- 3 cups cake flour

- 3 tablespoons lime juice

- 3 teaspoons baking powder

- 4 eggs, lightly beaten

- Grated peel of 1 lime

- Powdered sugar (not necessary)

Directions:

1. Preheat your oven to 325 degrees.

2. Sift together the cake flour, baking powder and salt three times; set aside.

3. In the container of an electric mixer, beat the butter until creamy.
4. Slowly put in in the sugar, then beat at moderate speed for five minutes, scraping down the sides of the container every so frequently.

5. Put in the beaten eggs slowly and carry on beating for 5 more minutes. (The mixture will be thick and twofold in volume.)

6. Using a rubber spatula, progressively fold in ¼of the flour mixture into the batter. Then fold in of the milk. Repeat this pulse until all of the flour and the milk have been blended. (You will put in flour last.)

7. Fold in the lime peel and lime juice.

8. Pour the batter into a greased molded cake pan, smoothing the surface and slightly building up the sides.

9. Bake the cake for 45 to 55 minutes or until the top is golden and the sides are starting to pull away from the pan.

10. Take out of the oven and allow to cool for one to two minutes. Cautiously unmold.

11. Allow to cool to room temperature. Sprinkle with powdered sugar or serve with Ginger Anglaise Sauce.

Yield: 1 (12-inch) cake

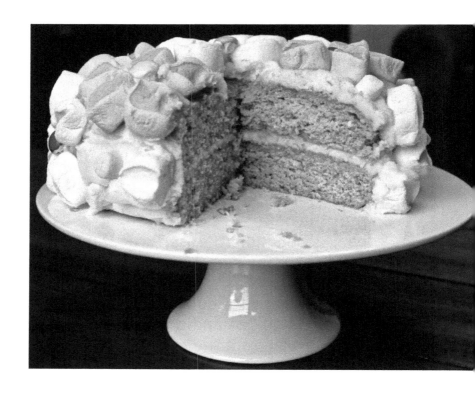

MANY PEAS ASIAN-STYLE SALAD

Ingredients:

- ½ cup fresh green peas

- ½ cup snow peas

- 1 cup sugar snap peas

- 1 tablespoon brown sugar

- 1 tablespoon rice vinegar

- 1 tablespoon sesame oil

- 2 teaspoons sesame seeds, toasted

- 2 teaspoons soy sauce

- 6 cups pea shoots or other sweet baby lettuce

Directions:

1. Bring a big pot of water to its boiling point. Put in the sugar snap peas and boil for a couple of minutes. Put in the snow peas and green peas and boil for a minute more. Drain and wash in cold water. Pat dry using paper towels.

2. In a big container, meticulously mix the sesame seeds, vinegar, oil, sugar, and soy sauce. Put in the peas and the greens and toss to coat.

Yield: Servings 4

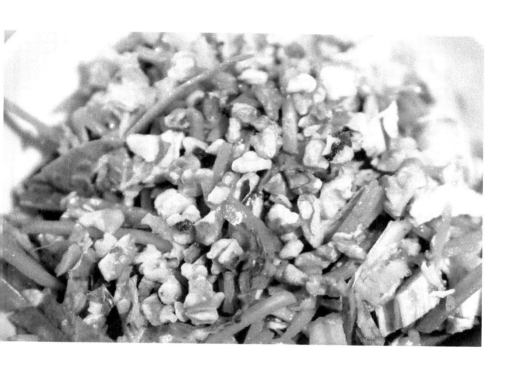

MARINATED MUSHROOMS

Ingredients:

- ¼ cup rice wine vinegar

- ½ cup water

- ¾ cup olive oil

- 1 whole serrano or jalapeño pepper

  1½ pounds whole small white
- mushrooms 2 stalks
- lemongrass

- 3 (½-inch) pieces gingerroot

- 3 cloves garlic

- Juice of 1 lime

Directions:

1. Put all of the ingredients apart from the mushrooms in a big pot; bring to its boiling point, reduce heat, and simmer for ten to fifteen minutes.

2. Put in the mushrooms to the pot, stirring to coat.

3. Take away the pot from the heat and let cool completely, approximately 1 hour.

4. Place in your fridge for minimum 2 hours, if possible overnight.

Yield: 25–35

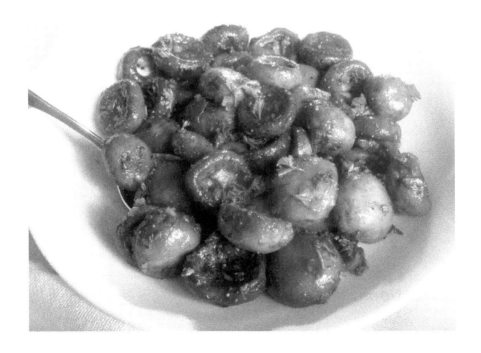

MERINGUES WITH TROPICAL FRUIT

Ingredients:

- 2 cups heavy cream, whipped

- 2 cups mixed fresh tropical

- 2 cups superfine sugar

- 6 egg whites

- Butter at room temperature to prepare baking dishes fruit, cut
- into bite-sized pieces

Directions:

1. Preheat your oven to 200 degrees. Butter pieces of parchment paper cut to line 2 baking sheets.

2. Put the egg whites in a cold container. Beat until tender peaks form Put in the sugar and carry on beating until firm.

3. Using a pastry bag, pipe 3- to 4 -inch circles of meringue onto the readied baking sheets.

4. Bake for 90 to 1twenty minutes or until they are dry, ensuring not to let the meringues turn color. If the meringues aren't dry after 2 hours of baking, turn the oven off and let the meringues sit in your oven overnight.

5. Allow the meringues to cool to room temperature. Fill a pastry bag with the whipped heavy cream. Pipe cream into the center of the meringues. Top with tropical fruit before you serve.

Yield: Approximately 24

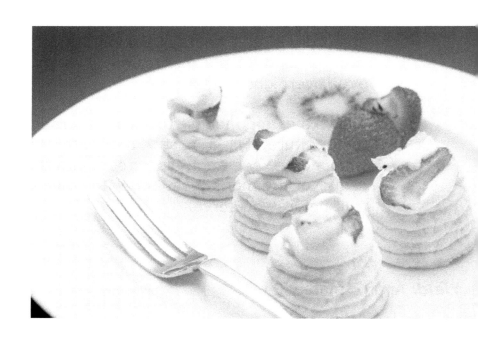

PEANUT-POTATO SALAD

Ingredients:

- ¼ cup chopped cilantro

- ¼ cup chopped mint

- ¼ cup peanut butter

- ¾ cup mayonnaise

- 1 cup salted peanuts, crudely chopped, divided

- 1 moderate-sized red bell pepper, cored and chopped

- 2 stalks celery, cut

- 3 pounds peeled boiling potatoes

- 3 tablespoons rice vinegar

- 4 green onions, trimmed and cut

- Salt and pepper to taste

Directions:

1. Bring a big pot of water to its boiling point using high heat. Put in the potatoes and cook until soft. Drain and cool. Cut into ½-inch cubes.

2. In a big container, mix the potato cubes, ¾ cup of peanuts, red bell pepper, celery, green onion, cilantro, and mint.

3. In a small container, whisk together the mayonnaise, peanut butter, and vinegar. Sprinkle salt and pepper to taste.

4. Pour the dressing over the potato mixture and toss to coat. Place in your fridge for minimum 1 hour. Decorate using the rest of the peanuts before you serve.

Yield: Servings 8–10

PICKLED CHINESE CABBAGE

Ingredients:

- 1 tablespoon chopped cilantro

- 1 tablespoon chopped garlic

- 2 big shallots or 1 medium onion, chopped

- 3 pounds Chinese cabbage, cored, halved, and thinly cut

- 4 cups water

- 6 cups rice vinegar

- Salt and white pepper

Directions:

1. Put all of the ingredients apart from the cabbage in a big stew pot and bring to its boiling point. Decrease the heat and simmer for five minutes.

2. Bring the cooking liquid back to its boiling point and mix in the cabbage. Cover and cook the cabbage for three to five minutes.

3. Take away the pot from heat and let cool completely. Season to taste with salt and white pepper.

4. Place in your fridge for minimum 8 hours before you serve.

Yield: 3 pounds

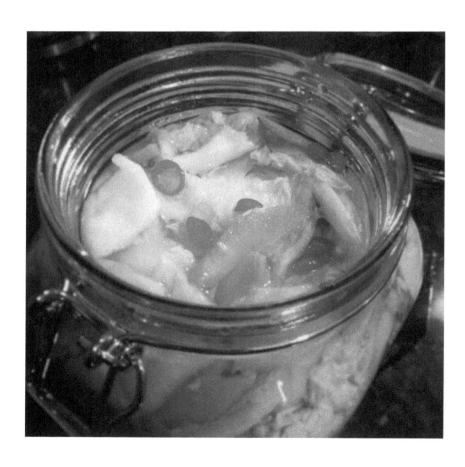

SOUTHEAST ASIAN ASPARAGUS

Ingredients:

- 1 cup toasted peanuts

- 1 pound asparagus, trimmed and slice into two-inch pieces

- 1 tablespoon sesame oil

- 1 teaspoon fish sauce

- 1 teaspoon toasted sesame seeds

Directions:

1. Heat the sesame oil in a big frying pan on moderate to high heat. Put in the asparagus and sauté for about three minutes.

2. Put in the fish sauce, sesame seeds, and peanuts. Sauté for two more minutes or until the asparagus is done to your preference.

Yield: Servings 4

SOUTHEAST ASIAN BURGERS

Ingredients:

- ¼ cup chopped basil

- ¼ cup chopped cilantro

- ¼ cup chopped mint

- 1 clove garlic, minced

- 1 pound ground beef or ground turkey

- 1 teaspoon sugar (not necessary)

- 2 tablespoons lime juice

- 3 shakes Tabasco

- 3 tablespoons bread crumbs

Directions:

1. In a moderate-sized-sized mixing container, mix all the rest of the ingredients.

2. Use your hands to gently mix the ingredients together and form 4 patties.

3. Season each patty with salt and pepper.

4. Grill the patties to your preference, approximately five minutes per side for medium.

Yield: Servings 4

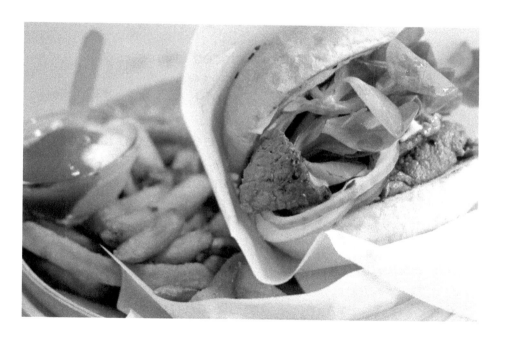

SPICY SHRIMP DIP

Ingredients:

- ½ serrano chili, seeded and minced
- ½ teaspoon grated lemon zest
- ½ teaspoon salt
- 1 tablespoon minced chives
- 5 tablespoons butter
- 8 ounces shrimp, cleaned and chopped
- Salt and freshly ground black pepper to taste

Directions:

1. In a moderate-sized-sized sauté pan, melt the butter on moderate heat. Mix in the chives, salt, chili pepper, and lemon zest; sauté for a couple of minutes.

2. Lower the heat to low and put in the shrimp; sauté for about three minutes or until opaque.

3. Move the mixture to a food processor and crudely purée. Sprinkle with salt and pepper.

4. Firmly pack the purée into a small container. Cover using plastic wrap, and place in your fridge for 4 hours or overnight.

5. To serve, remove the shrimp dip from the fridge and let it sit for five to ten minutes. Serve the dip with an assortment of crackers and toast points or some favorite veggies.

Yield: Approximately 1 cup

THAI CHICKEN PIZZA

Ingredients:

- ¼— cup peanut or hot chili oil

  ½ cup crudely chopped
  dry-roasted peanuts 1
- cup chopped cilantro
- leaves

- 1 medium carrot, peeled and crudely grated

- 1 recipe Asian or Thai Marinade

- 1 unbaked pizza crust

- 1½ cups bean sprouts

- 1½ cups fontina cheese

- 1½ cups mozzarella cheese

Directions:

1. Put the chicken breasts in an ovenproof dish.
   Pour the marinade over the chicken, flipping
   to coat completely. Cover and place in your
   fridge for minimum 8 hours. Allow the

chicken to return to room temperature before proceeding.

2. Preheat your oven to 325 degrees. Bake the chicken for thirty to forty minutes or until thoroughly cooked. Take away the chicken from the oven and let cool completely. Shred the chicken into minuscule pieces; set aside.

3. Prepare the pizza dough in accordance with package directions.

4. Brush the dough with some of the oil. Top the oil with the cheeses, leaving a ½-inch rim. Evenly spread the chicken, green onions, carrot, bean sprouts, and peanuts on top of the cheese. Sprinkle a little oil over the top.

5. Bake in accordance with package directions for the crust. Remove from oven, drizzle with cilantro, before you serve.

Yield: 1 large pizza

THAI PASTA SALAD

Ingredients:

- ¼ teaspoon ground ginger

- ½ teaspoon red pepper flakes

- 1 clove garlic, minced

- 1 cup bean sprouts

- 1 cup rice wine vinegar

- 1 tablespoon brown sugar

- 1 tablespoon soy sauce

- 1½ cups thinly cut Napa cabbage or bok choy 1½
- cups thinly cut red
- cabbage 2 medium
- carrots, shredded

- 2 tablespoons vegetable oil

- 2 tablespoons water

- 3 green onions, trimmed and thinly cut

- 3 tablespoons smooth peanut butter

- 8 ounces dried bow tie or other bite-sized pasta

Directions:

1. Cook the pasta in accordance with package directions. Drain and wash under cold water. Put the pasta in a big mixing container and put in the green onions, carrots, and cabbage.

2. In a small mixing container, meticulously mix all the rest of the ingredients except the sprouts.

3. Pour the dressing over the pasta and vegetables; cover and place in your fridge for minimum 2 hours or overnight.

4. Just before you serve, throw in the bean sprouts.

Yield: Servings 8–12

THAI-FLAVORED GREEN BEANS

Ingredients:

- ½ cup chopped cilantro

- 1 rounded tablespoon shrimp paste

- 2 pounds French or regular green beans, trimmed and slice into bite-sized pieces

- 2 tablespoons vegetable oil

- 2 teaspoons minced garlic

- 3 tablespoons unsalted butter

Directions:

1. In a pot big enough to hold all of the beans, steam them until soft-crisp.

2. Drain the beans, saving for later cooking liquid. Cover the beans using foil to keep warm.

3. In a small container, whisk together the shrimp paste and vegetable oil.

4. In a big frying pan, melt the butter on moderate to high heat. Put in the garlic and sauté until golden. Mix in the shrimp paste

mixture and 1 tablespoon of the reserved cooking liquid.

5. Put in the reserved green beans, stirring to coat. Cook until thoroughly heated.

6. Take away the pan from the heat and toss in the cilantro.

Yield: Servings 6–8

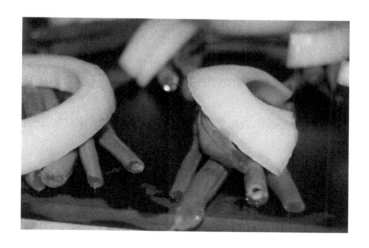

THAI-SPICED GUACAMOLE

Ingredients:

- 1 big plum tomato, seeded and chopped

- 1 small garlic clove, minced

- 1 tablespoon chopped onion

- 1 teaspoon chopped serrano or jalapeño chil

- 1 teaspoon grated gingerroot

- 1 teaspoon grated lime zest

- 1–2 tablespoons chopped cilantro

- 2 ripe avocados, pitted and chopped

- 4 teaspoons lime juice

- Salt and freshly ground black pepper to taste

Directions:

1. Put the avocado in a moderate-sized container. Put in the lemon juice and crudely mash.

2. Put in the rest of the ingredients and gently mix together.

3. Serve within 2 hours.

Yield: 2 cups

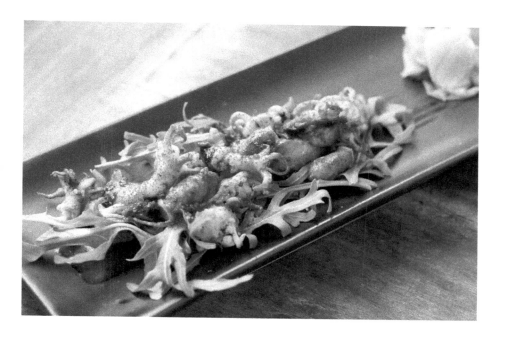

THAI-STYLE GRILLED PORK CHOPS

Ingredients:

- 1 cup fish sauce

- 2 (1-inch-thick) pork chops

- 2 tablespoons cream sherry

- 2 teaspoons brown sugar

- 2 teaspoons minced gingerroot

- 3 tablespoons rice vinegar

- garlic clove, minced

Directions:

1. In a small deep cooking pan, on moderate heat, bring the garlic, fish sauce, sherry, vinegar, brown sugar, and gingerroot to its boiling point. Turn off the heat and let cool to room temperature. (You can also put the marinade in your fridge to cool it.)

2. Put the pork chops in a plastic bag and pour in the marinade, ensuring to coat both sides of the chops. Allow the chops marinate at room temperature for fifteen minutes.

3. Pour the marinade into a small deep cooking pan and bring to a simmer on moderate to low heat. Cook for five minutes.

4. Grill the chops on a hot grill for five to six minutes per side for medium.

5. Serve the chops with the marinade sprinkled over the top.

Yield: Servings 2

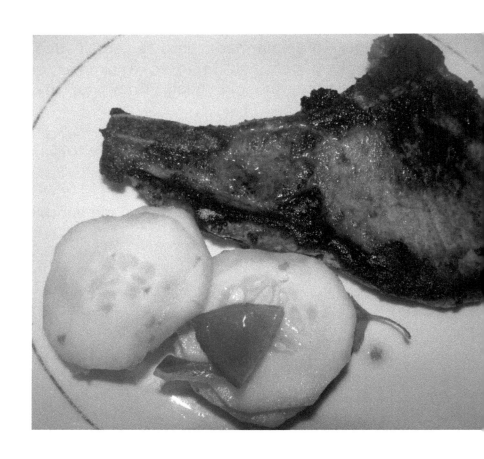

5 SPICED VEGETABLES

Ingredients:

- ¼ teaspoon crushed red pepper flakes

- ½ — ¾ teaspoon Chinese 5-spice powder

- ½ cup orange juice

- 1 cup carrot slices

- 1 pound mushrooms, cut

- 1 small onion, halved and thinly cut

- 1 tablespoon cornstarch

- 1 tablespoon vegetable oil

- 1–2 cloves garlic, minced

- 2 tablespoons soy sauce

- 2 teaspoons honey

- 3 cups broccoli florets

Directions:

1. In a small container, mix the orange juice, cornstarch, 5-spice powder, red pepper flakes, soy sauce, and honey; set aside.

2. Heat the vegetable oil in a wok or frying pan on moderate to high heat. Put in the mushrooms, carrots, onion, and garlic. Stir-fry for roughly 4 minutes.

3. Put in the broccoli and carry on cooking an extra 2 to 4 minutes.

4. Mix in the sauce. Cook until the vegetables are done to your preference and the sauce is thick, roughly two minutes.
5. Serve over rice noodles, pasta, or rice.

Yield: Servings 4

Lightning Source UK Ltd.
Milton Keynes UK
UKHW020724161222
414034UK00017B/1292